I0706801

THE WEALTH KNOWLEDGE OF HICCUPS

QUEST FOR A SOLTION FOR CHRONIC HICCUPS

Contents

Preface

This book presents an in-depth book written by esteemed experts in the field of hiccups. It offers a comprehensive examination of hiccups, covering various aspects such as their physiology, causes, and available treatment options.

The book begins by introducing hiccups as a common physiological occurrence and delves into their historical background and social importance. It outlines the aims and structure of the book, providing readers with a reasonable guide to what to expect.

The physiology of hiccups is totally explored, revealing insight into the anatomical and neurological aspects involved. Readers will acquire experience with the role played by the diaphragm, phrenic nerves, and brainstem in hiccup reflexes. In addition, the book explores the impact of neurotransmitters and neuronal pathways in hiccup mechanisms.

The causes and triggers of hiccups are explained in details, covering many variables that can cause hiccups. This includes gastrointestinal issues, emotional stress, temperature changes, and medication side effects. The book also examines the connection between hiccups and underlying medical conditions, such as strokes, brain tumors, and central nervous system disorders.

To aid in diagnosis, the book presents various diagnostic approaches, including physical examinations, medical history assessments, and potential imaging techniques. It emphasizes the importance of accurate diagnosis and distinguishes hiccups from similar conditions.

Management and treatment options for hiccups are thoroughly explored. Readers will discover a comprehensive range of strategies, including home remedies, behavioral techniques, and non-pharmacological interventions. The book also covers pharmacological options, such as medications targeting the central nervous system. Emerging therapies, including nerve stimulation are discussed as potential future directions.

The psychological and social impact of hiccups is another important aspect addressed in the book. It examines the effects of chronic hiccups on quality of life, emotional well-being, and interpersonal relationships. The book also provides insights into coping mechanisms and psychological support available for individuals affected by hiccups.

Looking towards the future, the book highlights ongoing research efforts and potential advancements in hiccup studies. It discusses the latest developments in medical technology and explores potential therapeutic innovations. The importance of interdisciplinary collaboration is emphasized for further understanding and progress in the field of hiccups.

The book concludes with an epilogue that shares personal stories and experiences of individuals living with chronic hiccups. It provides encouragement and support, summarizing key takeaways from the book, and emphasizing the significance of raising awareness about hiccups. Therefore, this book offers a comprehensive and authoritative resource for medical professionals, researchers, and individuals seeking a deep understanding of hiccups and the various aspects surrounding them.

Writing a book that has such a comprehensive scope requires wide consultation with various authorities and sources of information. I gratefully acknowledge friends and colleagues who contributed meaningful insights that enriched the book, especially the authors of published works whose materials formed the essential body of knowledge that this book builds on.

UNDERSTANDING THE BASICS OF HICCUPS

Introduction

Over the years, the study of hiccups has captivated researchers and medical professionals for a significant period of time. Despite being a common phenomenon experienced by almost everyone, hiccups present an intriguing puzzle that continues to spark scientific curiosity and investigation.

One reason hiccups have accumulated attention is their complicated nature. While hiccups are widely recognized, the exact cause and mechanisms behind their occurrence remain somewhat tricky. This knowledge gap has prompted researchers to investigate the basic physiological and neurological processes that lead to hiccups.

Moreover, hiccups can manifest in different forms and durations. Most hiccups are transient and resolve all by themselves; however, in some cases, they can persist for extended periods, causing distress and discomfort. Chronic hiccups, although moderately uncommon, can significantly affect a person's quality of life. This has motivated researchers to dive deeper into understanding the factors that contribute to the persistence of hiccups and exploring effective treatment options.

Furthermore, hiccups have been linked to a range of triggers and potential underlying medical conditions. Exploring the connection between hiccups and these factors has not only advanced our understanding of hiccup mechanisms but also given us experience in the wider context of human physiology and pathology.

The study of hiccups has profited from advancements in medical technology and imaging techniques. These tools have enabled researchers to observe and analyze hiccup-related phenomena in additional detail, uncovering complicated associations inside the nervous system and identifying likely focuses for therapeutic interventions.

Collaborative efforts between researchers from various disciplines, including neurology, gastroenterology, and respiratory medicine, have contributed to a comprehensive understanding of hiccups. This multidisciplinary approach has enriched the exploration of hiccups and has facilitated the development of diverse treatment modalities.

The study of hiccups has fascinated researchers and medical professionals due to the enigmatic nature of this common phenomenon. The quest to unravel the underlying mechanisms, explore triggers and associated conditions, and develop effective treatments has driven ongoing research efforts. Through interdisciplinary collaboration and advancements in technology, the study of hiccups continues to offer valuable insights into human physiology, ultimately aiming to improve the management and well-being of individuals affected by hiccups.

Therefore, hiccups as a common physiological phenomenon, are involuntary contractions of the diaphragm muscle, which plays a crucial role in the breathing process. They are experienced by almost everyone at some point in their lives and typically resolve spontaneously within a short period.

Hiccups are characterized by a sudden, involuntary "hic" sound produced due to the abrupt closure of the vocal cords during a contraction of the diaphragm. These contractions cause the characteristic jerking or spasm-like movement of the abdomen. While hiccups may seem like a trivial occurrence, they have captured the curiosity of researchers and medical professionals due to their intriguing nature. Despite their widespread occurrence, the exact cause of hiccups remains somewhat elusive.

Hiccups can be triggered by various factors. Gastrointestinal issues, such as overeating, swallowing air, or irritation of the diaphragm or phrenic nerves, are commonly associated with hiccups. Other triggers can include changes in temperature, excitement or emotional stress, certain medications, and underlying medical conditions affecting the central nervous system.

The duration of hiccups can vary. Most hiccups are short-lived and resolve on their own within minutes or hours. However, in some cases, hiccups can become persistent or chronic, lasting for extended periods and causing significant discomfort and disruption to daily activities. Chronic hiccups are less common but can be associated with underlying medical conditions or medications.

The study of hiccups involves exploring their underlying mechanisms, including the neurological pathways and muscles involved in hiccup reflexes. Researchers have also investigated the role of specific neurotransmitters, such as gamma-aminobutyric acid (GABA), in regulating hiccup mechanisms.

Understanding hiccups is not only of scientific interest but also holds practical significance. Researchers and medical professionals aim to develop effective treatments for persistent or chronic hiccups, as they can significantly impact an individual's quality of life.

Overview History of Hiccups

The phenomenon of hiccups, or involuntary contractions of the diaphragm muscle, has been known and experienced by humans for a long time. While the precise historical details are not extensively recorded, references to hiccups suggests that they have been observed and mentioned in various cultures throughout history.

Ancient civilizations had their own interpretations and explanations for hiccups. For instance, ancient Egyptian beliefs credited hiccups to the presence of evil spirits or demons, while ancient Greeks related them to divine intervention. These cultural beliefs often led to the development of rituals and practices aimed at dispersing hiccups, which were viewed as undesirable or even harmful.

To battle hiccups and avert the evil spirits or demons causing them, the ancient Egyptians developed rituals and practices. These rituals often involved particular actions or incantations performed by priests or other people knowledgeable in spiritual matters. By performing these rituals, they aimed to drive away the evil spirits and reestablish the normal functioning of the body, thereby stopping the hiccups.

Similarly, in ancient Greek culture, hiccups were related to divine intervention. It was believed that hiccups were caused by the impedance of the gods or other supernatural powers. The Greeks saw hiccups as a disturbance of the natural order and an indication of divine displeasure or intervention in the individual's life.

To address hiccups and appease the divine powers believed to be responsible, the ancient Greeks likewise developed their own rituals and practices. These practices often involved seeking divine favor through prayers, offerings, or performing particular actions to check the hiccup-initiating divine intervention. By doing so, they hoped to restore harmony and eliminate the hiccups caused by the divine powers.

In both ancient Egyptian and Greek cultures, the cultural beliefs surrounding hiccups led to the development of rituals and practices aimed at dispersing hiccups. These practices were attributed to the belief that hiccups were caused by extraordinary or spiritual impacts and were considered bothersome or possibly harmful. The rituals and practices were filled in for the purpose of restoring normalcy and balance, thereby resolving the hiccup peculiarity and eliminating any related worries or fears. Throughout history, old stories and superstitions surrounding hiccups have emerged in various cultures. People developed a range of remedies and techniques to try to stop hiccups. These remedies varied broadly and often had cultural or regional importance. Holding one's breath, drinking water in specific ways (such as from the far side of a glass or drinking while bending forward), or receiving sudden fright or surprise were commonly suggested methods to halt hiccups. Additionally, folk remedies such as swallowing sugar, breathing into a paper bag, or pulling on the tongue have been practiced in different cultures as well.

While hiccups have a rich cultural history, the scientific understanding of hiccups has advanced in recent times. Hiccups are now known to occur due to involuntary spasms of the diaphragm muscle, which plays a crucial role in breathing. These spasms result in the characteristic "hic" sound. Various factors can trigger hiccups, including rapid consumption of food or drink, ingestion of carbonated beverages, sudden temperature changes, emotional stress, or certain underlying medical conditions.

In most cases, hiccups are transient and self-limiting, resolving on their own without requiring any specific treatment. However, chronic or persistent hiccups that last for an extended period may indicate an underlying medical issue and may warrant medical attention to identify and address the underlying cause.

Anatomical and Neurological Aspects of Hiccups

From a neurological perspective, hiccups involve a complex interplay between the brain, the phrenic nerves, and the diaphragm muscle. The phrenic nerves originate from the spinal cord in the neck and innervate the diaphragm. They carry signals from the brain to the diaphragm, controlling its contraction and relaxation during breathing.

When hiccups occur, the brain sends abnormal signals to the diaphragm, leading to its involuntary contraction. This contraction happens abruptly and disrupts the normal rhythm of breathing. The diaphragm is a dome-shaped muscle located below the lungs, and it plays a crucial role in the process of respiration.

Normally, the diaphragm contracts and relaxes in a coordinated way, allowing us to easily breathe. However, during hiccups, this coordination is disrupted. The brain, especially the brainstem, which is involved in regulating essential body functions, plays a vital role in initiating and controlling hiccups.

The specific cause of the abnormal signals sent to the diaphragm during hiccups isn't fully understood, but It is believed that different triggers can stimulate certain nerves or centers in the brainstem, causing this abnormal signaling.

When the diaphragm contracts involuntarily, it pulls down and causes an unexpected intake of air into the lungs. Simultaneously, the closure of the vocal cords occurs, resulting in the trademark "hic" sound. This closure is a protective reflex to prevent a sudden or unexpected rush of air from entering the vocal cords, just like when we hold our breath or swallow.

The sudden closure of the vocal cords, along with the diaphragm contraction, creates the distinct sound associated with hiccups. This sound is the result of the air being removed from the closed vocal cords, making them vibrate and producing the hiccup noise.

It is worth noting that hiccups are usually transitory and resolve spontaneously within a short period of time. However, in some cases, hiccups can persist for a lengthy period or become chronic. Persistent or chronic hiccups might indicate a hidden medical condition or neurological disorder that requires further evaluation and treatment.

THE CAUSES AND TRIGGERS OF HICCUPS

Gastrointestinal Issues

Gastrointestinal issues such as acid reflux, swallowing air, or irritation of the diaphragm from overeating can lead to hiccups; and in response to this, we will be discussing how these conditions can trigger hiccups. Without wasting much time, lets delve in.

Acid reflux, which is also known as gastroesophageal reflux disease (GERD), occurs when the stomach acid and partially digested food flow back up into the esophagus. The esophagus is the tube that carries food from the mouth to the stomach. This backflow of stomach contents into the esophagus is known as acid reflux and can irritate the diaphragm, which is in close proximity to the lower part of the esophagus. This irritation of the diaphragm can trigger the hiccup reflex.

The lower esophageal sphincter (LES) is a ring of muscle located at the junction of the esophagus and the stomach. Its primary function is to act as a barrier, preventing stomach acid and food from regurgitating back into the esophagus. However, in some cases, the LES may weaken or relax inappropriately, allowing stomach acid to escape into the esophagus.

This weakening of the LES can be caused by various factors, such as *hiatal hernia* which occurs when a portion of the stomach protrudes through the diaphragm into the chest cavity. This can disrupt the normal functioning of the LES, making it more prone to opening and allowing acid reflux.

Excess weight and abdominal fat is another factor which can put pressure on the stomach, leading to increased chances of acid reflux. Additionally, it may contribute to a weakened LES.

Another factor is the intake of *Certain foods and drinks* which can relax the LES or stimulate the production of stomach acid, increasing the risk of acid reflux. Common triggers include spicy foods, fatty or fried foods, citrus fruits, tomatoes, chocolate, coffee, and alcohol.

During *pregnancy*, hormonal changes can relax the LES, making pregnant women more susceptible to acid reflux.

When stomach acid enters the esophagus, it can cause irritation, inflammation, and a burning sensation known as heartburn. In some cases, acid reflux can also lead to other symptoms such as regurgitation, difficulty swallowing, chest pain, and chronic cough.

Treatment for acid reflux may include lifestyle modifications such as dietary changes, weight management, avoiding trigger foods, and elevating the head of the bed during sleep. Although there are medications that can also be used to reduce stomach acid production and relieve symptoms, but in more severe cases, surgical interventions may be considered to strengthen the LES or repair a hiatal hernia.

Swallowing air, a condition known as aerophagia, can indeed lead to hiccups. When we swallow, it is normal to ingest a small amount of air along with saliva or food. However, excessive swallowing of air can occur due to various factors, such as eating or drinking too quickly, talking while eating, chewing gum, or consuming carbonated beverages.

When excess air accumulates in the stomach, it can cause distension and irritation. This irritation can stimulate the diaphragm, the muscle responsible for breathing, and lead to a hiccup reflex.

Swallowing air-induced hiccups are typically short-lived and resolve on their own. However, if aerophagia becomes a frequent or chronic issue, it may be necessary to address the underlying causes. Modifying eating habits, avoiding carbonated drinks, and practicing mindful eating can help reduce the swallowing of excess air and minimize the occurrence of hiccups associated with aerophagia.

Irritation of the diaphragm from overeating can also lead to hiccups. As we discussed earlier, the diaphragm is a large muscle that separates the chest cavity from the abdominal cavity and plays a significant role in the breathing process.

When we eat, especially if we eat a large amount of food in a short period, the stomach expands to accommodate the ingested food. This expansion can put pressure on the diaphragm, causing it to become irritated. The irritation of the diaphragm can trigger the hiccup reflex, resulting in the characteristic spasms of the diaphragm muscle and the accompanying hiccup sound.

Overeating can be a common cause of hiccups, especially when it leads to excessive stretching and irritation of the diaphragm. Hiccups in these cases are often temporary and subside as the stomach empties and the diaphragm returns to its normal state.

To prevent hiccups from overeating, it can be helpful to practice mindful eating, eat smaller and more frequent meals, and avoid overindulging in large quantities of food. Additionally, giving the body time to digest between meals and not lying down immediately after eating can help reduce the likelihood of hiccups associated with overeating.

Emotional Stress

When we experience strong emotions like anxiety, excitement, or stress, it can stimulate the nerves involved in the hiccup reflex. The hiccup reflex is a complex series of actions that involve several nerves in the body, particularly those associated with the respiratory system.

The hiccup reflex begins with the activation of the phrenic nerve, which originates from the neck and travels down to the diaphragm muscle, the primary muscle responsible for breathing. The phrenic nerve carries signal from the brain to the diaphragm, coordinating its contractions and relaxation during the breathing process.

During moments of intense emotions, the body undergoes physiological changes. These changes can include an increased heart rate, rapid breathing, and changes in the pattern of breathing. These alterations in breathing patterns can disrupt the normal coordination of the diaphragm muscle.

It is believed that the stimulation of the nerves involved in the hiccup reflex occurs due to the alteration in the pattern of breathing and the subsequent disruption in the coordination of the diaphragm muscle. This can lead to spasms or contractions of the diaphragm, resulting in hiccups.

The exact mechanisms by which emotions trigger the hiccup reflex are not fully understood and may vary among individuals. Emotional stress-induced hiccups are usually temporary and tend to resolve on their own as the emotional state stabilizes.

Managing and reducing emotional stress through various techniques such as deep breathing exercises, meditation, mindfulness, and seeking support from loved ones or professionals can help alleviate stress-related hiccups. If hiccups persist or become chronic, it is recommended to consult a healthcare professional for further evaluation and guidance.

Temperature Changes

While the exact mechanisms behind hiccups are still in progress, it is believed that temperature changes can potentially trigger hiccups due to their effect on the body's sensory receptors and nerve pathways.

When the body experiences sudden or extreme temperature changes, it can initiate specific reflex responses to maintain its internal balance and protect itself. These reflexes are designed to ensure the body's temperature stays within a narrow range and prevent any potential harm.

Temperature-related reflexes, such as the cold shock response or the activation of the trigeminal nerve (which senses facial sensations including temperature), may interfere with the normal rhythmic contractions of the diaphragm, leading to hiccups.

Furthermore, temperature changes can also affect the sensory receptors in the throat and esophagus. These receptors play a role in regulating swallowing and respiratory functions. Disruptions to these functions can potentially trigger hiccups as well.

It's important to note that not everyone experiences hiccups from temperature changes, and individual susceptibility may vary. Hiccups are generally temporary and harmless, and they typically resolve on their own without the need for medical intervention.

Medication Side Effects

Medication side effects can sometimes be a factor that also triggers hiccups. Although hiccups are typically temporary and benign, but certain medications can potentially disrupt the normal functioning of the diaphragm or the nervous system, leading to hiccups as a side effect; and below are some factors related to medication use that can contribute to hiccups:

Medications that affect the central nervous system: Certain medications that act on the central nervous system, such as benzodiazepines, opioids, or barbiturates, may have hiccups listed as a possible side effect. These medications can affect the normal coordination of the diaphragm and respiratory muscles, leading to hiccups.

Gastrointestinal medications: Some medications used to treat gastrointestinal conditions, like proton pump inhibitors (PPIs), can sporadically cause hiccups as a side effect. The specific component behind this isn't well understood yet, but it is believed to be related to the effect on the nerves and muscles of the digestive system.

It's vital to take note that medication-induced hiccups are commonly transient and resolve once the medicine is stopped, adjusted, or changed. If you experience persistent or bothersome hiccups as a side effect of medication, it is advisable to consult your healthcare provider. They can evaluate the situation, consider alternative medications if appropriate, or provide additional management strategies for the hiccups.

THE CLASSIFICATION OF HICCUPS

While hiccups are a common phenomenon, there has been ongoing research to study and classify them based on various factors. Classification systems help in understanding the characteristics, causes, and appropriate management of different types of hiccups. Although there is no universally accepted classification system, researchers have proposed different approaches based on their duration and the underlying causes.

Research in this area aims to improve the understanding of hiccups, identify potential causes, and develop effective treatment strategies. However, due to the relatively harmless nature of most hiccups and the lack of standardized classification systems, we will only be discussing these three (3) major classifications in the following passages;

Transient Hiccups

Transient hiccups are the most well-known type of hiccup and normally last for a short period, ranging from a couple of minutes to a couple of hours. They are often referred to as "everyday" hiccups and are viewed as normal and harmless. Transient hiccups occur unexpectedly and resolve all by themselves with no particular treatment.

These hiccups are typically triggered by factors that irritate or stimulate the diaphragm and the nerves involved in its functioning. Common triggers include eating food or beverages too fast, swallowing air, sudden excitement, stress, or changes in temperature. These triggers can prompt spasms of the diaphragm muscle, causing the trademark hiccup sound.

The self-limiting nature of transient hiccups means that they usually resolve without any intervention. The hiccup reflex eventually subsides as the underlying irritation or stimulation diminishes. Many people find relief through natural remedies or simple techniques such as holding their breath, drinking water, or distracting themselves.

While transient hiccups are generally harmless, they can be temporarily disruptive or uncomfortable. However, they do not typically indicate any underlying medical condition or require medical attention. If someone experiences occasional transient hiccups, there is usually no cause for concern.

If hiccups persist for an extended period, become frequent, or are accompanied by other concerning symptoms, it may be advisable to consult a healthcare professional. They can evaluate the situation, identify any underlying causes or contributing factors, and provide appropriate guidance or treatment if needed.

So, transient hiccups in general, are a common and temporary occurrence that does not usually require specific medical intervention.

Persistent Hiccups

Unlike transient hiccups, persistent hiccups are a type of hiccup that lasts for over forty-eight (48) hours but less than one month. They don't resolve immediately and may require medical intervention to reduce the symptoms and address any underlying causes.

While persistent hiccups are generally uncommon, they can be more disturbing and affect a person's day-to-day life. The prolonged duration of these hiccups often leads individuals to seek medical attention for alleviation.

Various underlying factors such as gastrointestinal issues, nerve irritation, and metabolic disorders like diabetes, kidney failure, or electrolyte imbalances can disrupt the normal functioning of nerves and muscles leading to persistent hiccups.

Additionally, certain medications such as steroids, benzodiazepines, or medications used for anesthesia, may have hiccups as a side effect.

To address persistent hiccups, medical professionals usually evaluate the underlying cause through a thorough medical history, physical examination, and potentially additional tests or imaging studies. Treatment options may vary depending on the identified cause and can include certain medications, such as muscle relaxants, anticonvulsants, or medications targeting the underlying condition, may be prescribed to alleviate persistent hiccups. But. in some cases, injecting an anesthetic or medication near the phrenic nerve can temporarily block its activity and provide relief from persistent hiccups.

Additionally, techniques like controlled breathing exercises, distraction methods, or swallowing maneuvers can help interrupt the hiccup reflex and give relief also.

Treating the underlying medical conditions or adjusting medications that might be causing hiccups can help resolve persistent hiccups. It is therefore important to consult a medical professional if you experience persistent hiccups or have worries about your symptoms. They can provide a proper evaluation, identify any underlying causes, and recommend suitable treatment options to ease the hiccups and improve your quality of life.

Intractable Hiccups

This is the most severe and persistent form of hiccups, lasting for more than one month. Unlike transient or persistent hiccups, intractable hiccups are extremely prolonged and can significantly affect a person's quality of life. They can cause physical discomfort, interfere with eating, sleeping, and speaking, and even lead to emotional distress and social embarrassment.

Identifying the specific underlying cause of intractable hiccups can be challenging, as numerous factors can contribute to their development. Some of these factors may include; conditions that affect the central nervous system, such as multiple sclerosis, brainstem lesions, encephalitis, or tumors located in or near the brainstem. These factors can disrupt the normal coordination of the muscles and nerves that are involved in hiccups, which would then result in intractable hiccups.

Certain metabolic disorders, such as liver or kidney failure, electrolyte imbalances, or diabetes, can also affect nerve and muscle function, including those involved in hiccupping.

In rare cases, other factors like medication, extreme stress, anxiety, or emotional trauma can also trigger or contribute to intractable hiccups. Addressing these factors through appropriate therapy or counseling may be necessary.

Given the chronic and debilitating nature of intractable hiccups, a comprehensive evaluation by healthcare professionals, including neurologists or specialists in gastroenterology, may be necessary. Diagnostic tests, such as imaging studies (MRI, CT scan), nerve conduction studies, or blood tests, may be performed to identify the underlying cause.

When hiccups become intractable, treating the underlying cause becomes crucial, and the treatment options for intractable hiccups can vary depending on the specific underlying cause. Prescription medications may be prescribed to help control the persistent hiccup reflex. But, in some cases, injecting an anesthetic or medication directly into the phrenic nerve or other nerve pathways involved in hiccupping can provide temporary relief.

Other options, like surgical procedures such as phrenic nerve diaphragmatic pacing or decompression surgeries for nerve compression, may be considered in severe and refractory cases. This option is usually very rare and uncommon.

In cases where psychological factors play a role, therapy or counseling to address underlying stress or emotional triggers may be beneficial.

The treatment approach for intractable hiccups should be tailored to the individual's specific situation and underlying cause. Close collaboration between healthcare professionals from different specialties may be necessary to manage and treat this challenging condition effectively.

THE DIAGNOSTIC APPROACHES FOR HICUPPS

The assessment of hiccups typically involves a thorough evaluation of the patient's medical history, a physical examination, and, in some cases, additional diagnostic tests. This diagnosis is primarily based on clinical evaluation and observation of the patient's symptoms, and there is no specific diagnostic test designed exclusively for hiccups. However, healthcare professionals may employ various methods, such as a combination of medical history, physical examination, and, in some cases, imaging techniques, to assess hiccups and determine any underlying causes or contributing factors.

There is no specific diagnostic test exclusively designed for hiccups because they are often transient and not indicative of an underlying serious medical condition. Hiccups are generally viewed as a physiological response and are often self-resolving without the need for thorough diagnostic processes.

During the clinical assessment, the healthcare provider will take a detailed medical history, including data about the characteristics of the hiccups (frequency, duration, triggers), related symptoms, and any factors that might worsen or alleviate the hiccups. They will likewise conduct a thorough physical examination to assess the patient's general well-being and look for any signs or symptoms that might suggest an underlying condition. In most cases, the diagnosis of hiccups depends on excluding other possible causes of persistent or intractable hiccups, like neurological disorders, gastrointestinal disorders, or metabolic abnormalities.

The absence of any significant findings during the medical history assessment and physical examination helps support the diagnosis of primary or benign hiccups. If the healthcare provider suspects an underlying condition contributing to the hiccups, further diagnostic tests may be ordered to investigate the specific cause. These tests are targeted at identifying and evaluating the suspected underlying condition rather than directly diagnosing hiccups themselves.

It's important to note that the vast majority of hiccups are temporary and benign, resolving spontaneously without medical intervention. Treatment for hiccups is typically focused on managing any underlying causes or triggers, if identified, and providing symptomatic relief.

Now, let's explore each of these diagnostic methods in more details.

Medical History Assessment

A thorough medical history assessment plays a vital role in understanding a patient's hiccups and identifying potential basic causes or triggers. It involves gathering detailed data about the patient's previous medical history, current symptoms, lifestyle factors, and any other significant details. **Current Symptoms:** During assessment, the healthcare provider will pose specific inquiries about the hiccups, including the frequency, duration, and pattern of occurrence. They will investigate when the hiccups began, how long they last, and whether they happen spontaneously or are triggered by specific factors. Details about the sound, intensity, and any related symptoms, such as pain, agony, or difficulty breathing, are important to note.

Medical History: Subsequent to assessing the current symptoms, the healthcare provider will then ask about the patient's previous medical history, including any chronic conditions, past surgeries, or critical illnesses. Certain medical conditions, like gastroesophageal reflux disease (GERD), diabetes, neurological disorders, or respiratory conditions, can be related to hiccups. A history of any past episodes of hiccups or similar symptoms may likewise be significant.

Medications: A review of the patient's current medications, including prescription drugs, non-prescription medications, and herbal supplements, is significant. Some medications can trigger hiccups as a side effect and changes in medication regimens or the ongoing initiation of new medications ought to be noted.

Lifestyle Factors: The healthcare provider will also inquire about the patient's lifestyle habits and factors that may be associated with hiccups. This includes dietary habits, such as eating spicy or hot foods, consuming carbonated beverages, or rapid eating. Alcohol consumption, smoking history, stress levels, and recent changes in daily routines or emotional state can also be potential triggers or exacerbating factors.

Associated Symptoms: The provider will also, explore any associated symptoms that accompany the hiccups, such as chest pain, abdominal discomfort, difficulty swallowing, or changes in bowel movements. These associated symptoms may provide important clues about underlying conditions or complications related to the hiccups.

Red Flags: This involves the healthcare provider to be vigilant for any red flags or warning signs that may suggest a more serious underlying cause of hiccups. Symptoms such as unexplained weight loss, severe or persistent pain, neurological deficits, difficulty speaking or swallowing, or respiratory distress require further investigation and may warrant additional diagnostic tests.

By conducting a comprehensive medical history assessment, the healthcare provider can gather pertinent information and clues that aid in understanding the hiccups and determining their underlying cause. This information helps guide further diagnostic evaluation or direct appropriate management strategies to provide relief to the patient.

It's important for patients to provide accurate and detailed information during the medical history assessment, as even seemingly unrelated details can be relevant in identifying the triggers or causes of hiccups. Clear communication and collaboration between the patient and healthcare provider are essential for an accurate assessment and effective management of hiccups.

Physical Examination

During a physical examination for hiccups, the healthcare professional will thoroughly assess different regions of the body to identify any potential hidden medical conditions that could be related to the hiccups. The following is a breakdown of the explanation.

Head and Neck Examination: The healthcare professional will inspect the head and neck region, checking for any abnormalities or signs that could contribute to hiccups. They might inspect the cranial nerves, palpate the neck for lymph nodes or masses, and examine the throat, tonsils, and oral cavity for any indications of inflammation, infection, or underlying abnormalities.

Chest Examination: The chest will be examined to assess the respiratory system and check for any abnormalities that could be linked to hiccups. The healthcare professional might pay attention to the lungs for abnormal breath sounds, evaluate the respiratory efforts, and assess the chest wall for possible injuries or indications of injury.

Abdominal Examination: Here, the healthcare expert will carry out a thorough examination of the abdomen to evaluate the gastrointestinal system and distinguish any possible causes of hiccups. They will palpate the abdomen to check for tenderness, organ extension, masses, or indications of inflammation. Specific attention might be given to the diaphragm area, as irritability or dysfunction of this muscle can lead to hiccups.

Neurological Examination: A neurological examination is often done as hiccups can be related to nervous system dysfunction. The healthcare professional will evaluate the patient's reflexes, muscle strength, coordination, and sensation. They may likewise assess cranial nerves, including the vagus nerve, which plays a role in the hiccup reflex.

Depending on the patient's symptoms and suspected basic causes, additional regions of the body might be examined. For instance, if there are signs or symptoms suggestive of spinal cord or peripheral nerve involvement, the healthcare professional might evaluate the spine and extremities and perform explicit neurological tests.

By evaluating the head, neck, chest, abdomen, and other important body regions, the healthcare professional aims to identify any abnormalities, indications of irritation, injury, or masses that could be contributing to the hiccups. These discoveries, along with the patient's medical history and other diagnostic tests, help guide further investigation and the management of the hiccups.

It's essential to take note that the physical examination is tailored to the individual patient's case, and not all components might be important in each circumstance. The healthcare professional will focus on relevant areas based on the patient's symptoms, medical history, and suspected basic causes.

Potential Imaging Techniques

When evaluating hiccups and potential underlying causes, healthcare professionals might utilize different imaging techniques to get detailed visual data about particular organs or structures. These imaging techniques play a significant role in identifying underlying abnormalities, tumors, or other conditions that might be contributing to the hiccups. Here are some common imaging techniques used in this context.

X-rays: These utilize ionizing radiation to make images of the body's internal structures. While not often used for investigating hiccups directly, they can be useful in evaluating the chest and diaphragm for abnormalities like lung diseases, cracks, or indications of respiratory conditions that could be related to hiccups.

Computed Tomography (CT) Scan: CT scans combine X-rays and PC technology to create detailed cross-sectional images of the body. CT scans give more detailed data than X-rays and can help identify possible causes of hiccups in different body regions. For instance, CT scans of the chest, abdomen, or head can reveal abnormalities like tumors, infections, or underlying issues that might contribute to hiccups.

Magnetic Resonance Imaging (MRI): MRI uses strong magnetic fields and radio waves to create detailed images of the body's inner structures. It provides great soft tissue visualization and is specifically helpful for examining the central nervous system, including the brain and spinal cord. MRI can help identify neurological causes of hiccups, like brain tumors, vascular mutations, or other abnormalities.

Ultrasound: Ultrasound imaging utilizes high-frequency sound waves to make images of organs and tissues. It is generally used for assessing the abdomen, including the liver, gallbladder, kidneys, and gastrointestinal tract. Ultrasound can help identify any underlying abnormalities or organ dysfunction that might be related to hiccups.

Endoscopy: This involves inserting a thin, flexible tube with a light and camera into the body to visualize and examine internal organs or cavities. Upper gastrointestinal endoscopy or bronchoscopy may be performed to evaluate the upper digestive tract or airways if there is suspicion of abnormalities contributing to hiccups. These procedures can help identify conditions like gastroesophageal reflux disease (GERD), esophageal disorders, or respiratory tract abnormalities.

The choice of imaging technique depends on the suspected underlying cause of hiccups and the specific areas of the body being investigated. The healthcare professional will determine the most appropriate imaging modality based on the individual patient's symptoms, medical history, and physical examination findings. These imaging techniques provide valuable information that aids in accurate diagnosis and guides appropriate treatment for the underlying cause of hiccups.

Evaluating Tools for Hiccups

The evaluation of hiccup intensity and its effect on quality of life can be facilitated by using diagnostic criteria and questionnaires. These tools help healthcare professionals evaluate the features and severity of hiccups, as well as their impact on an individual's everyday activities and well-being. While hiccups are generally viewed as a harmless condition, persistent and severe hiccups can significantly influence a person's quality of life, and it is essential to properly evaluate and address them.

Diagnostic criteria are standard guidelines that assist healthcare professionals in making accurate diagnoses. In spite of the fact that there is no universally accepted set of diagnostic criteria for hiccups, some systems have been proposed to help with evaluating hiccup severity. For instance, the "Chicago Classification" is one such system used for evaluating chronic hiccups. It categorizes hiccups based on duration (acute vs. chronic), frequency (short bouts vs. continuous), and underlying cause (idiopathic vs. secondary to an identifiable medical condition). These criteria help differentiate between transient, self-limiting hiccups and persistent or pathological hiccups that may require further investigation and management.

Questionnaires are organized tools consisting of a series of questions and inquiries that individuals complete to provide data about their symptoms, experiences, and quality of life. With regards to hiccups, questionnaires can assist in capturing the emotional effect of hiccups on an individual's well-being. They might ask about the frequency, duration, and intensity of hiccups, as well as their interference with day-to-day activities, sleep disturbances, emotional distress, and social interactions.

One generally used questionnaire is the "Hiccup Impact on Daily Life" (HIDL) questionnaire. It is an approved tool intended to evaluate the effect of hiccups on quality of life. The HIDL questionnaire includes things related to physical discomfort, emotional health, social work, and the general effect of hiccups on day-to-day activities. By scoring the responses, healthcare providers can measure the severity of hiccups and their impact on an individual's quality of life.

Another questionnaire used in hiccup research is the "Alabama Quality of Life" (AQOL) questionnaire. Although not specific to hiccups, it is a general quality of life questionnaire that can be adapted to evaluate the impact of hiccups on various aspects of well-being.

Both diagnostic criteria and questionnaires play complementary roles in evaluating hiccup severity and its impact on quality of life. Diagnostic criteria provide a structured framework for categorizing hiccups based on their characteristics and potential underlying causes, while questionnaires capture the subjective experience and functional impairment caused by hiccups. Integrating both approaches allows for a comprehensive assessment of hiccups and informs appropriate management strategies to improve the individual's quality of life.

THE MANAGEMENT AND TREATMENT OPTIONS FOR HICCUPS

Hiccups, although typically harmless and short-lived, can indeed be bothersome when they persist or significantly affect a person's quality of life. Fortunately, there are various management strategies that can be employed to alleviate or eliminate hiccups, the following passages are several approaches that can help:

Holding Your Breath

Taking a deep breath and holding it is a method commonly suggested to relieve hiccups. The diaphragm, which is a dome-shaped muscle situated between the chest and the abdomen, plays a significant role in the process of breathing by contracting and relaxing to assist with inhalation and exhalation.

When you take a deep breath and hold it, you create a temporary pause in your normal breathing pattern. This break in the breathing cycle can help regulate the diaphragm and possibly stop hiccups. It is believed that the act of holding the breath stimulates the vagus nerve, which is linked to the diaphragm and controls its movement.

This vagus nerve is a significant nerve that runs from the brainstem through the neck, chest, and abdomen, and it plays a crucial role in regulating different body functions, including breathing. By stimulating the vagus nerve, you can impact the activity of the diaphragm and possibly interfere with the hiccup reflex.

When you hold your breath, it can cause an increase in carbon-dioxide levels in the bloodstream. This change in the blood's composition might help regulate the diaphragm's constrictions and reset its normal beat, effectively stopping the hiccups.

It's important to take note that while holding your breath can be effective for some individuals, it may not work for everybody, particularly in persistent or chronic cases of hiccups. If hiccups persist or significantly affect your quality of life, seeking medical attention for further evaluation and the right management is advisable.

Drinking Water or Swallowing

Sipping cold water or swallowing a teaspoon of sugar are common remedies suggested to interrupt the hiccup reflex by stimulating the vagus nerve. The vagus nerve, also known as the cranial nerve X, is a long nerve that extends from the brainstem down through the neck, chest, and abdomen. It is involved in regulating various bodily functions, including digestion, heart rate, and breathing.

When you sip cold water or swallow sugar, it triggers a sensory response in the throat and mouth. This sensory stimulation can activate the vagus nerve, which has branches that innervate these areas. The activated vagus nerve sends signals to the brain, specifically the part responsible for coordinating the diaphragm and other respiratory muscles.

By stimulating the vagus nerve, you can potentially interrupt the hiccup reflex, which involves involuntary contractions of the diaphragm. It is believed that this interruption can help reset the diaphragm's rhythm and stop the hiccups.

The exact mechanism behind why cold water or sugar may stimulate the vagus nerve and interrupt hiccups is not fully understood. However, it is thought that the sudden sensation of temperature or taste triggers a reflex response in the nerves of the throat and mouth, leading to the activation of the vagus nerve and subsequent modulation of the diaphragm's activity.

It's important to note that while sipping cold water or swallowing sugar can be effective for some people, the response may vary among individuals. If hiccups persist or become chronic, it is advisable to consult with a healthcare professional for further evaluation and appropriate management.

Pulling Knees to Chest

The method you mentioned, sitting on the edge of a seat, leaning forward, and pulling your knees toward your chest, is believed to help stretch the diaphragm and possibly stop hiccups. As discussed earlier, the diaphragm is a large muscle situated underneath the lungs, separating the chest cavity from the abdomen cavity. It plays a major role in the process of breathing.

When you sit on the edge of a seat and lean forward, you create a position that urges the diaphragm to stretch and expand. By pulling your knees toward your chest, you further elongate the middle part of the body and make more space for the diaphragm to move.

The idea behind this method is that stretching the diaphragm helps direct its regulation and contractions, which can interrupt the hiccup reflex. Hiccups happen when the diaphragm contracts involuntarily and spasmodically. By elongating and stretching the diaphragm, you may be able to reset its rhythm and stop the hiccups.

Additionally, assuming this position can also create a change in your body's overall posture and muscle tension, potentially affecting the nerve impulses and signals related to hiccups. It's possible that the altered position and stretching may help reset the diaphragm's activity and relieve hiccups.

It's important to note that while this technique can be effective for some individuals, it may not work for everyone, especially in persistent or chronic cases of hiccups. If hiccups persist or significantly affect your quality of life, it is advisable to seek medical attention for further evaluation and appropriate management.

Gargling with Ice Water

Gargling with cold water is another method that is believed to stimulate the nerves toward the back of the throat and possibly interrupt on the hiccup reflex.

When you gargle with cold water, the sensation of the cool temperature triggers a reflex reaction in the nerves situated at the back of your throat. These nerves are part of the glossopharyngeal nerve, one of the cranial nerves involved with the swallowing and gag reflex.

The act of gargling with cold water activates these nerves, which are associated with the brainstem. This stimulation can send impulse to the brain, possibly affecting the diaphragm's activity and interfering with the hiccup reflex.

The specific mechanism by which gargling with cold water hinders hiccups isn't totally understood. However, it is believed that the stimulation of the glossopharyngeal nerve and its association with the central nervous system can trigger a response that influences the rhythmic contraction of the diaphragm, leading to the end or cessation of hiccups.

It means a lot to take note of that while gargling with cold water can be effective for certain individuals, individual responses might vary.

It may not work for everyone or in persistent or chronic cases of hiccups. If hiccups persist or significantly impact your quality of life, it is advisable to consult with a healthcare professional for further evaluation and appropriate management.

Pressure Points

Applying pressure to specific points on the body, such as the palm of the hand or the area between the eyebrows, is also a technique that is believed to help relieve hiccups. These points are associated with acupressure, which is a practice derived from traditional Chinese medicine.

According to acupressure principles, the body has energy pathways called meridians, and certain points along these meridians are believed to have specific effects when pressure is applied to them. In the case of hiccups, applying pressure to certain points may help restore balance and alleviate the spasms of the diaphragm.

The palm of the hand and the area between the eyebrows are two commonly suggested acupressure points for hiccups:

Palm of the hand: The palm contains several acupressure points, and pressing or massaging these points may help interrupt the hiccup reflex. The exact points recommended can vary, but generally, they are found in the center of the palm or near the base of the thumb. Applying firm but gentle pressure or massaging in a circular motion on these points is suggested.

Area between the eyebrows: This point is known as the "Yintang" or "Third Eye" point in traditional Chinese medicine. It is located between the eyebrows, at the spot where the bridge of the nose meets the forehead. Applying gentle pressure to this point or massaging it in a circular motion is believed to have a calming effect on the nervous system, potentially helping to alleviate hiccups.

The mechanism behind why applying pressure to these points may relieve hiccups is not well understood from a scientific standpoint. It is thought that the pressure or stimulation of these specific points may activate nerves or release certain substances in the body that can influence the diaphragm's spasms and interrupt the hiccup reflex.

While acupressure techniques can be helpful for some individuals in relieving hiccups, it is important to also note that scientific evidence supporting their effectiveness is limited. The response to acupressure can vary among individuals, and it may not work for everyone or in persistent or chronic cases of hiccups.

Distraction Techniques

Engaging in activities that divert your attention is another technique often recommended to interrupt the hiccup cycle and alleviate hiccups. The underlying idea is that hiccups can be influenced by the central nervous system, and by focusing your attention on something else, you can disrupt the reflex arc responsible for hiccups.

When you divert your attention, especially by engaging in mentally challenging activities, it can shift the focus away from the hiccups and help interrupt the hiccup cycle. Counting backward from a specific number, solving a puzzle, or engaging in any task that requires concentration can occupy your mind and potentially break the pattern of hiccups.

By mentally redirecting your attention, you may be able to override the reflexive contractions of the diaphragm and reset its rhythm. This technique can be effective for some individuals, particularly in cases where hiccups are triggered by stress, anxiety, or other psychological factors.

The exact mechanism behind how diverting attention helps alleviate hiccups is not fully understood. However, it is believed that by engaging in mentally stimulating tasks, you activate different neural pathways and circuits in the brain, which can modulate the activity of the diaphragm and potentially interrupt the hiccup reflex.

It's important to note that while diverting attention can be helpful for many people, individual responses may vary. Additionally, this technique may not be effective in persistent or chronic cases of hiccups. It is therefore advisable to consult a healthcare professional for further evaluation and appropriate management if your hiccups persist or significantly affecting your quality of life.

Medications

In persistent cases of hiccups, when other management strategies have not been effective, a doctor may consider prescribing medications to help control the spasms of the diaphragm. These medications can include muscle relaxants, sedatives, or medications that affect the nervous system.

Muscle relaxants that can help reduce the spasms of the diaphragm work by inhibiting the nerve signals that cause the muscles to contract involuntarily. These medications can be effective in managing persistent or chronic hiccups by relaxing the diaphragm and restoring its normal rhythm.

Certain sedative medications, may be prescribed to help calm the nervous system and interrupt the hiccup reflex. Sedatives can have a relaxing effect on the diaphragm and other muscles involved in breathing, potentially reducing hiccup frequency and intensity.

Medications that affect the nervous system, may also be used to modulate nerve activity and regulate the diaphragm's contractions. These medications work by altering the transmission of certain neurotransmitters involved in the hiccup reflex, helping to break the cycle of hiccups.

It's important to note that the use of these medications for hiccups is typically reserved for persistent cases that significantly affect a person's quality of life and have not responded to other management strategies. The specific medication and dosage will depend on the individual's medical history, underlying conditions, and other factors, and should be determined by a healthcare professional.

Additionally, it's worth mentioning that some medications may have potential side effects or interactions with other drugs, so it's essential to follow the healthcare professional's instructions and discuss any concerns or questions with them.

THE IMPACT OF HICCUPS

Psychological Distress

While hiccups are basically harmless and transient, lasting only a few minutes to a few hours, chronic hiccups, which are referred to as hiccups that persist for more than 48 hours or recur frequently over an extended period, often lasting weeks or even months, can lead to several mental and social consequences, such as psychological distress.

Unlike ordinary hiccups that typically resolve on their own, persistent hiccups can be highly frustrating and irritating despite various attempts to stop them, such as holding breath, drinking water, or other common remedies. This inability to control or stop the hiccups can lead to feelings of weakness and a deficiency of control over one's own body, which can be distressing.

The continuous nature of chronic hiccups can create anxiety and emotional strain. Individuals might experience increased anxiety due to the uncertainty of when the hiccups will stop or, on the other hand, if they will at any point go away. This chronic condition of anxiety can unavoidably affect one's general well-being, leading to increased stress levels and emotional pressure. The steady disturbance caused by the hiccups can create a sense of unpredictability in day-to-day activities, as individuals might never know when the next hiccup episode will happen. This unpredictability can contribute to feelings of distress as individuals are continually tense, anticipating the next hiccup and its possible effect on their activities and interactions.

The frustration and distress related to chronic hiccups can negatively affect mental health. The prolonged disturbance and inconvenience can gradually wear down an individual's strength, leading to feelings of irritability, agitation, and even anger. The steady presence of the hiccups can create a huge distraction, making it hard for individuals to focus on tasks or enjoy activities they usually find pleasurable. This disturbance in day-to-day life can further contribute to a decreased sense of well-being and overall fulfillment.

Moreover, the psychological distress caused by chronic hiccups can have a cascading effect on other parts of an individual's life. Sleep disturbances are common with persistent hiccups, as the hiccup might go on all night, making it difficult to get enough sleep. Sleep deprivation can worsen psychological distress, affecting mood, cognitive function, and general mental health.

It is crucial to acknowledge the psychological effects of chronic hiccups and offer help to individuals experiencing this condition. Seeking medical evaluation and exploring treatment options can be crucial not only in managing the physical symptoms but also in addressing the psychological distress associated with chronic hiccups. Psychological interventions such as counseling or therapy may be beneficial in helping individuals cope with emotional challenges and develop strategies to improve their overall well-being.

Anxiety and Depression

As the constant interruption of day-to-day activities by the hiccup can be frustrating and disappointing, individuals might experience anxiety as they anticipate the next hiccup and the effect it will have on their ability to perform tasks or take part in social interactions. The vulnerability about when the hiccups will stop or if they will ever go away can create a sense of increased anxiety and worry.

This can likewise lead to sleep deprivation, further fueling anxiety. The hiccup episodes can persist during sleep, causing continuous awakenings or keeping individuals from falling asleep in the first place. Sleep deprivation can fundamentally affect mental health, as it can impede cognitive function, increase irritability, and elevate emotional reactivity. The lack of getting enough sleep due to chronic hiccups can contribute to a state of chronic anxiety and further reduce an individual's overall mood and quality of life.

Over time, the chronic anxiety associated with chronic hiccups can contribute to the development or exacerbation of depressive symptoms. The ongoing stress and emotional strain of living with persistent hiccups can wear down an individual's resilience and coping mechanisms. Feelings of sadness, hopelessness, and a decreased sense of enjoyment in activities that were once pleasurable can emerge. The chronic disruption caused by hiccups can create a sense of despair, as individuals may struggle to see a way out of the condition and feel trapped in their hiccup state. These depressive symptoms can further contribute to a diminished quality of life and overall well-being.

It is crucial to address the emotional toll of chronic hiccups alongside the physical symptoms. Seeking medical attention and exploring treatment options can be helpful in managing both the hiccups themselves and the associated anxiety and depressive symptoms. Healthcare professionals can provide support, offer strategies for coping with anxiety, and, if necessary, refer individuals to mental health professionals who can provide counseling or therapy to address the psychological impact of chronic hiccups.

Social Embarrassment and Self-esteem

Chronic hiccups can really be socially embarrassing especially for individuals experiencing them. The repetitive hiccup sound, which may be louder or more frequent than ordinary hiccups, can draw attention to the person. The involuntary jolting of the body that usually goes with hiccups can likewise be noticeable and add to the social embarrassment.

The likely interruption of discussions or social interactions due to hiccups can further contribute to self-consciousness. Hiccups can interrupt one's speech or make it challenging to communicate effectively, causing frustration and hindering the flow of conversation. This interruption can lead to a fear of being judged or ridiculed by others, as the hiccups might be seen as uncommon or abnormal.

The social embarrassment related to chronic hiccups can fundamentally affect an individual's self-esteem. Persistent hiccups can cause individuals to have a self-conscious outlook on their appearance, their capacity to control their bodies, or their general sense of normalcy. They might not feel quite the same as others or worry that they will be seen as strange or odd. These feelings of disgrace, shame and self-consciousness can reduce self-esteem as time goes on, leading to a negative self-image and a reduced sense of self-worth. The fear of social embarrassment and judgment can likewise contribute to a reluctance to engage in social activities. Individuals with chronic hiccups might avoid social gatherings, public events, or even close relationships due to the discomfort, distress, and anxiety related to the condition. This social withdrawal can lead to feelings of isolation, depression, loneliness and a sense of being disconnected from others. The avoidance of social interactions can further fuel feelings of social anxiety and sustain a cycle of isolation.

It is important to offer help and understanding to individuals experiencing chronic hiccups. Establishing a tolerant and compassionate environment can help alleviate and lighten the social embarrassment and self-esteem issues they might face. Encouraging open communication about the condition and promoting education and awareness can also help reduce stigma and misconceptions surrounding chronic hiccups. Additionally, seeking medical evaluation and exploring treatment options can help manage the hiccups and potentially alleviate the social challenges associated with them.

Occupational and Educational Functioning

The disruptive nature of chronic hiccups, characterized by unexpected and involuntary interruptions, can make it difficult to concentrate and maintain focus on an individual's ability to perform day-to-day activities, including work and education. These interruptions caused by hiccups can disrupt workflow and hinder productivity.

Constantly stopping or repeating activities due to hiccups can lead to inefficiency and delays in finishing work or tasks. It can likewise make it hard to sustain sustained mental effort, as the hiccup episodes can act as distractions and break the continuity of concentration. As a result, individuals with chronic hiccups might experience decreased productivity and weakened performance. They might struggle to meet deadlines or accomplish the level of quality in their work that they want or that is required of them. This can lead to increased work-related pressure or stress, as individuals might feel disappointed and frustrated by their powerlessness to perform at their best due to the persistent hiccups.

The negative impact of chronic hiccups on work or education can extend beyond individual assignments or tasks. It can affect overall work fulfillment and professional advancement. If chronic hiccups continue over a long period of time, they can limit professional growth opportunities or hinder performance assessments. The disturbances caused by hiccups may likewise affect interpersonal relationships in the workplace or study hall, as individuals might struggle to fully engage in teamwork, conversations, or presentations.

In educational settings, chronic hiccups can slow down learning and academic advancement. Students may find it challenging to focus during lectures, participate in classroom activities, or complete exams and assignments without interruptions. The persistent hiccups can hinder comprehension, retention, and the ability to concentrate during study sessions.

Generally, chronic hiccups can contribute to work-related stress, decreased job satisfaction, and potential negative impacts on career advancement or academic progress. It is essential for individuals experiencing chronic hiccups to seek medical attention and explore treatment options to manage the condition effectively. By addressing the hiccup episodes, individuals can regain the ability to concentrate, focus, and perform daily tasks more efficiently, thus minimizing the impact on their professional and educational pursuits.

The Ongoing Research and Its Advancement

The ongoing research efforts in hiccup studies focus on understanding the mechanisms, exploring potential treatments, and investigating the neurological basis of hiccups. Hiccups are thought to originate from a reflex arc that involves several components, including the phrenic and vagus nerves, as well as the central pattern generator in the brainstem.

While the involvement of the phrenic and vagus nerves and the central pattern generator in hiccups is well-established, the exact neural pathways and brain regions responsible for hiccup generation are still being investigated. Future research aims to elucidate the precise mechanisms underlying hiccups by examining the interactions between these components and identifying the specific neural circuits involved.

Neuroimaging techniques, such as MRI and EEG, are valuable tools for studying the brain regions and neural networks associated with hiccup generation. By observing brain activity during hiccups, researchers can identify the specific brain regions that are activated or inhibited during these episodes. This information helps in understanding how hiccup-related neural circuits are organized and how they function. Additionally, animal models, such as rodents, have been used to study the neural mechanisms. By recording neural activity in these animal models during hiccup-like events, researchers can gain insights into the neural circuits and pathways involved.

Therefore, ongoing research in understanding the precise mechanisms underlying hiccups aims to further unravel the neural basis of hiccups, identify the specific neural pathways involved, and shed light on the complex interplay between the phrenic and vagus nerves, the central pattern generator, and other brain regions associated with hiccup generation.

It also is focused on identifying triggers and underlying causes beyond the well-known factors. By investigating potential connections between hiccups and conditions such as gastrointestinal disorders, central nervous system disorders, metabolic abnormalities, and psychological factors, researchers aim to gain a better understanding of the mechanisms through which these conditions contribute to hiccup generation. This research may ultimately lead to improved diagnostic approaches and more targeted treatments for hiccups associated with specific underlying causes or medical conditions.

Importance of Interdisciplinary Collaboration for Further Research

Interdisciplinary collaboration plays a crucial role in furthering our understanding of hiccups. Hiccups are a complex physiological phenomenon that involves various systems and processes in the body. It encompasses both physiological and neurological aspects, requiring insights from different fields such as neuroscience, physiology, pharmacology, gastroenterology, psychology, and biomedical engineering. Each discipline brings a unique perspective and expertise to the study of hiccups, allowing for a more comprehensive understanding of the phenomenon.

The neuroscience explores the neural mechanisms underlying hiccups. Neuroscientists investigate the neural pathways, brain regions, and neurotransmitter systems involved in hiccup generation. They use techniques such as neuroimaging, electrophysiology, and optogenetics to identify and study the neural correlates of hiccups. Their insights help unravel the intricate neural circuitry and the functional interactions between different brain regions during hiccup episodes.

While Physiologists contribute by examining the physiological processes involved in hiccups. They study the muscular activity, particularly of the diaphragm and other respiratory muscles, during hiccup episodes. Physiological measurements help identify the changes in muscle contractions, breathing patterns, and associated physiological responses that occur during hiccups. Their findings provide insights into the physiological mechanisms underlying hiccup generation and regulation.

The Pharmacologists investigate the effects of various medications and drugs on hiccups. They study the pharmacological agents that can modulate the neural pathways and neurotransmitter systems involved in hiccup generation. Through preclinical and clinical trials, they evaluate the efficacy and safety of pharmacological interventions for hiccups. Their research helps identify potential drug targets and develop targeted medications to alleviate hiccups.

Gastroenterologists explore the relationship between hiccups and gastrointestinal disorders. They investigate how conditions such as gastroesophageal reflux disease (GERD), hiatal hernia, or esophagitis can trigger or contribute to hiccups. Gastroenterologists study the anatomical and functional connections between the digestive system and the hiccup reflex. Their expertise helps identify the potential gastrointestinal triggers and provides insights into the interaction between the gut and hiccup generation.

Psychologists contribute by examining the psychological factors that may influence hiccups. They study the impact of emotional stress, anxiety, or psychological states on hiccup episodes. Psychologists explore the role of the autonomic nervous system and the mind-body connection in hiccup generation. Their insights help understand the psychological factors that can modulate the frequency and severity of hiccups and inform the development of behavioral and cognitive techniques for hiccup management.

Biomedical engineers contribute by developing innovative devices and technologies for hiccup management. They design and optimize therapeutic devices that can deliver targeted stimulation or provide sensory feedback to interrupt the hiccup reflex. Biomedical engineers also collaborate with other disciplines to develop advanced imaging techniques, wearable sensors, and data analysis methods that aid in studying hiccups. Their expertise facilitates the translation of research findings into practical applications for hiccup diagnosis, monitoring, and treatment.

By integrating insights from these diverse fields, interdisciplinary collaboration enhances our understanding of hiccups from multiple angles. It allows for a comprehensive examination of the physiological, neurological, pharmacological, psychological, and technological aspects of hiccups. Such collaboration promotes a more holistic approach to hiccup research and fosters the development of effective diagnostic tools, targeted therapies, and personalized interventions for individuals experiencing hiccups.

Living with Hiccups

Living with chronic hiccups can be incredibly challenging and disruptive to an individual's daily life. Chronic hiccups can persist for weeks, months, or even years, causing physical discomfort, social embarrassment, and psychological distress.

According to Sarah's story, she developed chronic hiccups after a severe bout of flu. Initially, she didn't think much of it, assuming they would disappear on their own. However, days turned into weeks, and her hiccups persisted relentlessly. Sarah tried different remedies recommended by friends and family, including drinking water, holding her breath, and even having someone scare her. Unfortunately, nothing seemed to work. The constant hiccups made it difficult for her to eat, sleep, and engage in normal conversations. She often found herself avoiding social gatherings and isolating herself due to embarrassment. It took several months of visiting different specialists and undergoing various medical tests until she finally found a treatment plan that helped alleviate her hiccups. While they haven't completely disappeared, they have significantly reduced, allowing her to regain some semblance of normalcy in her life.

Similar to Mark's story; His chronic hiccups started suddenly one evening while he was having dinner with his family. They thought it was a passing occurrence, but the hiccups persisted for days without relief. Mark's hiccups were not only physically exhausting but also mentally draining. He experienced constant fatigue from the energy expended during hiccup episodes, which made it difficult for him to focus on his work and daily tasks. He also struggled with sleeping due to the interruptions caused by hiccups throughout the night. The frustration and helplessness he felt took a toll on his mental well-being, leading to anxiety and depression. Mark sought medical assistance, trying different medications and therapies to alleviate his hiccups. It took a while, but eventually, with the help of a multidisciplinary approach involving medication, relaxation techniques, and counseling, he was able to manage his hiccups better and improve his quality of life.

These stories highlight the physical, emotional, and social impact chronic hiccups can have on individuals. It's important to remember that each person's experience is unique, and the severity and duration of chronic hiccups can vary. Seeking medical advice and support from healthcare professionals is crucial for managing chronic hiccups and finding effective treatment options.

Summary

Raising awareness about hiccups is important to increase understanding, support, and access to resources for individuals experiencing hiccups, particularly chronic hiccups. Chronic hiccups can have a significant impact on a person's physical and emotional well-being, disrupting daily activities, sleep, and social interactions. By raising awareness, we can promote empathy, reduce stigma, and encourage early recognition and diagnosis. Additionally, awareness initiatives can drive research efforts, leading to advancements in treatment options and improved quality of life for those affected by hiccups.

Raising awareness about hiccups is essential for creating a supportive environment, reducing the burden of chronic hiccups, and improving the overall well-being of individuals experiencing this condition. Through education, understanding, and research advancements, we can better support those affected by hiccups and enhance their quality of life.

A Message to Inspire you

Dear friend,

I want you to know that you are an inspiration. Living with chronic hiccups is no easy feat, yet here you are, facing each day with courage and resilience. Your strength in the face of this challenge is remarkable, and I want to encourage you to keep pushing forward.

I understand that chronic hiccups can be frustrating, exhausting, and at times, overwhelming. But please remember that you are not defined by this condition. You are a unique individual with dreams, passions, and a spirit that can't be dampened by hiccups.

Embrace your journey and the lessons it brings. Through this experience, you have gained a deep understanding of patience, empathy, and the strength of the human spirit. Your resilience serves as a shining example to others facing their own struggles.

While it may feel like a lonely road at times, know that you are not alone. Reach out to your loved ones, support groups, or online communities that can provide a listening ear and offer valuable advice. Sharing your story can bring comfort and may even inspire others who are going through similar challenges.

Remember to take care of yourself both physically and emotionally. Prioritize self-care and engage in activities that bring you joy and relaxation. Celebrate the small victories along the way, for each step forward is a testament to your strength and determination.

Never lose hope. Medical advancements are constantly being made, and with the support of healthcare professionals, you will find a treatment or management plan that works for you. Keep advocating for yourself, asking questions, and exploring different options. You deserve relief and a better quality of life.

You are capable of overcoming this obstacle, and I believe in your ability to find peace and happiness, regardless of the hiccups that may persist. Your journey is a testament to the incredible strength of the human spirit. Keep shining your light, inspiring others, and living life to the fullest.

With admiration and support,

From all of us @Med Spirit.